Pleasure Mastery

An Ultimate Guide to Satisfying Your Man in Bed

Cheryl Bach

Pleasure Mastery

Cheryl Bach

Table of Contents

Pleasure Mastery

Cheryl Bach

Introduction

Purpose of the Book

"Pleasure Mastery: An Ultimate Guide to Satisfying Your Man in Bed" is a comprehensive guide aimed at empowering women to take control of their sexuality and provide their male partners with a fulfilling and satisfying sexual experience. This book offers practical guidance, techniques, and advice that readers can use to enhance their lovemaking skills, increase their confidence in bed and achieve a more profound emotional and sexual connection.

Why Sexual Pleasure is Important in a Relationship

Sexual pleasure is a crucial element in maintaining a healthy, and thriving relationship. By prioritizing your partner's sexual satisfaction, you are creating an intimate space for growth, exploration, and vulnerability. This sends a powerful message to your partner that they are cherished, valued, and desired. Moreover, prioritizing your partner's sexual pleasure helps foster a deep level of trust and emotional connection between both partners.

Sexual pleasure can also have a positive impact on your physical health. Research shows that regular sexual activity can lead to improved sleep, reduced stress levels, a stronger immune system, and even lower blood pressure.

Why It's Important to be Proactive when it Comes to Sexual Satisfaction

Being proactive when it comes to sexual satisfaction means taking ownership of your own pleasure and actively investing in your relationship's sexual wellbeing. When you take the initiative to explore your sexuality, communicate your preferences and desires with your partner, and prioritize their sexual needs, you are contributing towards a healthy, fulfilling, and mutually beneficial sex life.

Taking an active role in your sexual satisfaction also fosters self-confidence and empowerment. It helps you to become more comfortable with your own body, desires, and preferences, empowering you to communicate your sexual needs confidently and assertively. This can lead to a deeper sense of personal fulfillment and a stronger sense of self-worth.

Being proactive also means being open and willing to try new things. This can involve trying out different sexual positions, role-playing scenarios, or experimenting with toys or lubricants. By exploring your sexuality in this way, both you and your partner can discover new ways to experience pleasure, which can ultimately strengthen your emotional connection.

In summary, the introduction of "Pleasure Mastery: An Ultimate Guide to Satisfying Your Man in Bed" emphasizes the importance of prioritizing sexual pleasure in a healthy relationship, and highlights the benefits of taking an active, proactive approach when it comes to achieving sexual satisfaction. In the following chapters, we will dive deeper into specific techniques, tips, and strategies to help you enhance your sexual experiences and achieve greater levels of intimacy and connection with your partner.

Chapter 1

Understanding the Male Anatomy

The Male Sexual Anatomy - An Overview

The male anatomy is complex, and understanding it is crucial to satisfying your man in bed. It's essential to know about the various structures and organs involved in sexual pleasure and how they function together.

The following is a brief overview of the male anatomy:

The Penis: The penis is the primary sexual organ in men, composed of three parts, the root, shaft, and glans. The head of the penis (glans) contains nerve endings that make it highly sensitive to touch, which makes it the primary site for sexual arousal.

The Testicles: The testes are two oval-shaped glands located in the scrotum. Their function is to produce sperm and male hormones such as testosterone. They're also an incredibly sensitive area, and many men enjoy having them touched or stimulated during sexual activity.

The Prostate Gland: The prostate gland is a small gland located below the bladder and in front of the rectum. It's responsible for producing fluid that helps transport sperm during ejaculation. The prostate gland can be stimulated through the anus, which can lead to intense orgasmic sensations.

Understanding Male Sexual Response

Understanding how men's bodies typically respond to sexual arousal can help you better understand how to satisfy your man in bed.

Men's sexual response generally occurs in four phases:

Excitement Phase: This phase is characterized by an increased heart rate, elevated blood pressure, and an erection. During this phase, men experience sexual arousal from physical touch, visual stimuli, or mental stimulation.

Plateau Phase: In this phase, the body continues to build tension, breathing becomes more rapid, and the testicles move closer to the body. Men may also experience pre-ejaculation or pre-cum during this phase.

Orgasmic Phase: This is the peak of sexual response, characterized by involuntary muscle contractions throughout the body and ejaculation. The intensity and duration of orgasms vary for each man.

Resolution Phase: In this final phase, the body returns to its resting state, with the penis returning to its flaccid state, and the heart rate and breathing slowing down.

Pleasure Mastery

It's important to remember that every man is different, and the timing and duration of each phase can vary. It's essential to communicate with your partner and understand their unique sexual response to help enhance their pleasure.

Tips on Exploring Your Partner's Anatomy

Exploring your partner's anatomy is a crucial step towards understanding what brings them pleasure and satisfying them in bed.

Here are some tips to help you explore your partner's anatomy:

Pay attention to their reactions: During sexual activity, pay attention to your partner's body language, breathing, and vocalizations. This can give you clues as to what they find pleasurable and what they don't.

Ask for feedback: Communication is key when it comes to sexual satisfaction. Don't be afraid to ask your partner if they're enjoying what you're doing or if there's something else they would like you to try.

Experiment with different touch and pressure: Try varying the pressure, speed, and location of your touch to see what feels best for your partner. You can also try using different parts of your body for stimulation, such as your lips or tongue.

Use lubrication: Lubrication can make stimulation more comfortable and pleasurable for both you and your partner. Experiment with different types of lubricants to find one that works best for both of you.

Try different positions: Different sexual positions can provide different levels of stimulation, so try experimenting with different positions to see what your partner enjoys.

Explore erogenous zones: The male body has many erogenous zones besides the obvious ones. Some of these zones may be unexpected, so spend time exploring different areas of your partner's body to see what they like.

Incorporate toys or props: Sex toys or other props can add an extra layer of stimulation to sexual activity. Again, communication is key, so make sure to discuss using toys with your partner beforehand.

Remember, the goal of exploring your partner's anatomy is not just to find what brings them physical pleasure but also what emotional and mental aspects of sex your partner enjoys. Your partner may have unique fantasies or desires, so be open to trying new things and exploring together.

Chapter 2

Mindset Shift

The Importance of Mindset in Great Sex

When it comes to sex, mindset and attitude play a crucial role in achieving great pleasure. If you're worried, stressed, or distracted, it can be difficult to be present and enjoy the moment fully. On the other hand, adopting a positive and open mindset can make all the difference in your sexual experiences.

Here's how:

Confidence: Being confident in your body and your desires can be incredibly attractive and powerful. When you feel confident in yourself, you're more likely to take charge in the bedroom and actively pursue what you want.

Trust and Vulnerability: Trust is a vital component of any sexual relationship. When you trust your partner and feel safe being vulnerable with them, you can let go of any inhibitions that may have been holding you back. This allows for a deeper level of intimacy and pleasure.

Presence: Being present in the moment means focusing on the sensations and experiences you're currently feeling rather than worrying about performance or past experiences. This can allow you to fully enjoy the moment and be mindful of your partner's needs and desires.

Tips for Shifting Your Mindset

If you struggle with negative thoughts or anxieties around sex, there are several tips that can help you shift your mindset towards pleasure:

Practice Self-Love: Spending time practicing self-love can help build confidence and create a positive attitude towards yourself and your sexual experiences. This can include practices such as meditation, journaling, or affirmations.

Focus on Sensations: Instead of focusing on achieving orgasm or meeting certain expectations, focus on the sensations and experiences you're feeling in the moment. Pay attention to the way your body feels and the sensations you're experiencing without trying to control or change them. This can help you let go of any expectations and fully enjoy the experience.

Communicate with Your Partner: Communication is key to great sex. Talk to your partner about your desires, boundaries, and fantasies. This can help you build trust and feel more comfortable being vulnerable with them. More open communication can lead to a deeper level of intimacy and pleasure.

Experiment: Trying new things can be invigorating and exciting. Experimenting with new positions, toys, or fantasies can help you explore your sexuality and desire. This can also lead to more open communication between you and your partner and can enhance your sexual experiences.

Encouragement to Explore Your Sexuality and Desire

Exploring your sexuality and desire is an important part of achieving pleasure mastery. However, it can be difficult to know where to start or to feel comfortable exploring your desires.

Here are some ways to encourage and support yourself in exploring your sexuality and desire:

Embrace Your Fantasies: Fantasies are a normal and healthy part of human sexuality. Instead of shaming yourself for having certain desires, embrace them and explore them in a safe and consensual way.

Seek Out Resources: There are many resources available to those looking to explore their sexuality and desires, such as books, podcasts, and online communities. Seek out resources that resonate with you and that can provide guidance and support.

Practice Self-Care: Exploring your sexuality and desires can be emotionally and mentally challenging. Make sure to prioritize self-care practices such as meditation, exercise, and spending time with loved ones to provide emotional support.

Take Your Time: Exploring your sexuality and desires is a journey, not a destination. Give yourself time to explore and experiment without putting pressure on yourself to have it all figured out right away.

Be Open-Minded: Keep an open mind when exploring new sexual experiences and desires. Being open-minded can lead to new and exciting experiences that you may not have considered before.

In conclusion, a positive mindset and attitude towards sex are essential for achieving pleasure mastery. By shifting your mindset towards pleasure, exploring your sexuality and desires, and communicating openly with your partner, you can create deeper levels of intimacy and pleasure in your sexual experiences. Remember that there is no one "right" way to experience pleasure, and the key is to focus on what feels good and enjoyable for you and your partner.

Chapter 3

Communication and Listening

The Importance of Communication and Active Listening

Effective communication and active listening are crucial components of any sexual relationship. Without them, it can be difficult to understand your partner's desires and needs, leading to unsatisfactory sexual experiences.

Here's why communication and active listening are so important:

Understanding Needs: Good communication allows you and your partner to understand each other's needs and desires, leading to more satisfying sexual experiences.

Building Trust: Trust is vital in any sexual relationship. Effective communication builds trust, creating a safe and comfortable environment to share fantasies and desires.

Resolving Conflicts: Conflicts can arise during sexual experiences. Effective communication can help you resolve conflicts and understand each other's boundaries.

Techniques for Initiating Conversations about Sexual Desires and Needs

Initiating conversations about sexual desires and needs can be challenging, especially if you are shy or uncomfortable discussing sensitive topics. However, it is essential for building intimacy and improving the quality of your sexual experiences.

Here are some techniques for initiating conversations about sexual desires and needs:

Create a Safe Space: Before initiating a conversation about sexual desires and needs, make sure that you are in a safe and comfortable environment. Create a non-judgmental and accepting space where both you and your partner feel comfortable expressing yourselves.

Start Small: It can be helpful to start with small questions or conversation starters to gauge your partner's interest and comfort level. For example, you might ask what their favorite sexual position is or what they enjoy most about sex.

Use "I" Statements: When discussing sexual desires and needs, it's important to use "I" statements instead of "you" statements. This means framing the conversation in terms of your own experiences and feelings, rather than blaming or accusing your partner. For example, instead of saying "You never do this for me," you might say "I really enjoy when we do X during sex."

Listen Actively: Active listening means being fully present and engaged in the conversation, without interrupting or judging your partner's thoughts or feelings. This means giving your partner your full attention and asking questions to clarify their perspective.

Be Open-Minded: Keep an open mind during the conversation about sexual desires and needs. Allow your partner to share their thoughts and feelings, even if they differ from your own. Try to understand their perspective and seek common ground.

The Role of Body Language in Communication during Sex

Body language plays a crucial role in communication during sex. Nonverbal cues can communicate desires, feelings, and needs without words. Understanding and responding to body language during sex can enhance intimacy and pleasure.

Here are some ways to use and interpret body language during sex:

Eye Contact: Eye contact is a powerful way to connect with your partner during sex. It communicates intimacy, trust, and desire. Maintaining eye contact during sexual activity can increase feelings of pleasure and connection.

Touch: Touching is a form of nonverbal communication that can communicate desire, comfort, and pleasure. Pay attention to how your partner responds to touch and adjust your actions accordingly.

Body Movements: Body movements can communicate pleasure and discomfort. Pay attention to your partner's body movements during sex to gauge what feels good and what does not.

Vocalizations: Moaning, groaning, and other vocalizations during sex can communicate pleasure and desire. Pay attention to the sounds your partner makes and adjust your actions accordingly.

Facial Expressions: Facial expressions during sex can communicate a range of emotions, from pleasure and desire to discomfort and pain. Look for signs of pleasure, such as a flushed face or dilated pupils, as well as signs of discomfort, such as a grimace or furrowed brow.

It's important to note that body language can vary from person to person, so it's essential to communicate openly with your partner about what feels good and what doesn't. Using body language in conjunction with verbal communication can enhance intimacy and pleasure, leading to a more satisfying sexual experience.

In conclusion, effective communication and active listening are crucial components of any sexual relationship. Initiating conversations about sexual desires and needs can be challenging, but following these techniques can help you and your partner build trust and intimacy. Understanding the role of body language in communication during sex can enhance intimacy and pleasure by allowing partners to better communicate their desires and needs without words.

Chapter 4

Foreplay

The Importance of Foreplay

Foreplay is often overlooked, but it is an important aspect of sexual pleasure and intimacy. Foreplay can help increase arousal, lubrication, and overall sexual satisfaction.

Here's why foreplay is so essential:

Increases Arousal: Foreplay helps to build anticipation and arousal, making sexual experiences more pleasurable.

Enhances Lubrication: Foreplay prepares the body for intercourse by increasing vaginal lubrication, making sex more comfortable and enjoyable.

Cheryl Bach

Improves Communication: Foreplay can be an opportunity to communicate with your partner about your desires, boundaries, and preferences.

Different Types of Foreplay

Foreplay can take many forms, from gentle touches to passionate kisses.

The different types of foreplay can include:

Kissing: Kissing is a classic form of foreplay that can be gentle or passionate, depending on your preferences.

Touching: Touching can involve gently caressing your partner's body, exploring their erogenous zones, and stimulating their genitals.

Oral Sex: Oral sex involves using your mouth, tongue, and lips to stimulate your partner's genitals. This can include both giving and receiving oral sex.

Pleasure Mastery

Dirty Talk: Dirty talk involves communicating your desires, fantasies, and preferences to your partner in a way that is sexually arousing.

Erotic Massage: Erotic massage involves using different techniques to massage your partner's body, focusing on their erogenous zones to increase arousal.

Roleplaying: Roleplaying involves acting out different scenarios or fantasies to explore your sexual desires and enhance intimacy.

Techniques to Bring Him to the Edge

Here are different techniques you can use during foreplay to bring your man to the edge of climax:

Tease him: You can build anticipation and arousal by teasing your man. This could include soft touches, whispering dirty talk into his ear, or playing with his erogenous zones.

Use your mouth: Oral sex can be an effective way to bring your man close to climax. Use your lips, tongue, and mouth to stimulate his penis, balls, and perineum.

Explore his body: Discover which parts of his body feel most sensitive and responsive. Pay attention to how he reacts when you touch certain areas, and adjust your technique accordingly.

Use sex toys: Incorporating sex toys such as vibrators, dildos, or cock rings can add even more excitement and pleasure to your foreplay.

Incorporate dirty talk: Talking dirty can set the mood and create a sense of intimacy. Use language that turns your man on, and share your fantasies with him.

Try edging: Edging involves bringing your man close to orgasm and then stopping stimulation just before he reaches the edge. This can prolong the pleasure and increase the intensity of the eventual orgasm.

Engage in mutual masturbation: Watching each other masturbate can be incredibly arousing. This can include touching and stimulating each other while masturbating or taking turns masturbating for each other.

Experiment with different positions: Changing positions during foreplay can keep things interesting and exciting. Experiment with different positions, locations, and techniques to find what works best for you and your partner.

In conclusion, foreplay is a crucial component of sexual pleasure, helping to build arousal, lubrication, and overall satisfaction. Understanding the importance of foreplay and incorporating different types of techniques during your sexual encounters can enhance intimacy and pleasure. By using your mouth, exploring your partner's body, incorporating toys, and trying different positions, you can bring your man to the edge and maximize sexual pleasure. Remember to communicate openly with your partner and pay attention to their body language to ensure a mutually satisfying experience. Don't underestimate the power of foreplay, it could be the key to unlocking mind-blowing orgasms!

Chapter 5

The Art of Oral Sex

Detailed Instructions on How to Give Pleasure with Oral Sex

Oral sex can be an incredibly intimate and pleasurable experience for both partners.

Here is a step-by-step guide on how to give pleasure with oral sex:

Prepare: Before you start, make sure you and your partner are clean and groomed. Take the time to set the mood, perhaps by lighting candles or playing music.

Start Slowly: Begin by kissing and softly licking your partner's inner thighs, slowly moving towards their genitals.

Use Your Tongue: Gently use your tongue to explore your partner's genitals. Try different techniques like using small circular motions around the glans, flicking the frenulum, or tracing the rim of the head with your tongue.

Build Intensity: After spending some time building up your partner's arousal, you can begin to take things up a notch by introducing new techniques and intensifying your movements. Use the flat part of your tongue to cover more surface area while gently licking, lightly suck on his penis, and use more pressure as he gets closer to orgasm.

Switch Things Up: Don't be afraid to switch up your techniques and try different movements or positions. Ask your partner what he likes and adjust your technique accordingly.

Pay Attention to His Reactions: Be aware of your partner's body language and vocalizations. This can help you understand what feels good for him and how to better satisfy him.

Communicate: Oral sex is a two-way street, so communicate with your partner about what you like and what you don't. This can help ensure a mutually satisfying experience.

Explanation of Techniques for Deep Throating, Using Your Tongue and Teeth

Deep throating, using your tongue and teeth can all be great techniques to incorporate into your oral sex sessions.

Here's how to do each one:

Deep Throating:

While deep throating is not necessary for pleasurable oral sex, it can be an enjoyable experience for both partners.

Follow these steps to safely deep throat:

Cheryl Bach

Start slow: Begin by taking just the head of his penis into your mouth and gradually work your way down.

Relax: When you feel ready to take more of his shaft, relax your throat muscles, inhale through your nose, and let his penis glide further into your mouth.

Control Your Breathing: If you feel like you're gagging, try swallowing or pausing to control your breathing before continuing to inhale and take more of his penis into your mouth.

Use Your Hands: To make it easier, use your hands to stroke his shaft while you focus on deep throating just the head.

Communicate: Communicate with your partner throughout the experience to ensure that you're both comfortable and enjoying it.

Using Your Tongue:

Using your tongue is a great way to add variety and pleasure to oral sex.

Here are some techniques to try:

Flat Tongue: Use the flat part of your tongue to cover as much surface area as possible, moving up and down his shaft or in circles around the glans.

Pointed Tongue: Use the tip of your tongue to tease and tickle the sensitive areas like his frenulum.

Flicking Tongue: Lightly flick your tongue along the rim of his head for added stimulation.

Twirling Tongue: Use your tongue to twirl around his penis in alternating directions, like a swirl.

Using Your Teeth:

Using your teeth can be a little bit tricky and requires careful attention to avoid causing any pain or discomfort.

Here are some techniques to try:

Lightly Nipping: Gently bite down on his penis with your teeth, using a light pressure that doesn't cause pain.

Teasing with Teeth: Use your teeth to lightly graze his shaft or head, creating a teasing sensation with the added texture.

Combining Techniques: You can also combine the use of your tongue and teeth for various sensations. For example, you can use your tongue to twirl around his head while lightly grazing it with your teeth.

Different Positions that Work for Oral Sex

Oral sex can be performed in a variety of positions, which can add to its excitement and intimacy.

Here are some positions to consider:

69: This is a classic position where both partners can pleasure each other at the same time. One partner lies on their back while the other positions themselves above them, each taking turns giving and receiving oral pleasure.

Sitting: In this position, the man can sit on the edge of a bed or chair, while the woman kneels in front of him. This position can provide a great angle for deep throating.

Lying Down: This can be performed with the man lying down on his back with his head propped up by a pillow, while the woman positions herself between his legs. This position can provide easy access to all parts of the penis.

Standing: In this position, the man stands while the woman kneels in front of him, providing a great angle for deep throating. This position can also add an element of dominance and submission to the experience.

Doggy Style: For this position, the woman can get on all fours and the man can kneel behind her, allowing her to pleasure him from this angle. This position can be fun and playful, as well as great for those who enjoy a little bit of kink.

Side by Side: In this position, both partners lie on their sides with the woman positioned between the man's legs. This can provide a more intimate and connected experience, as well as an easy angle for deep throating.

Remember, every couple is unique, and what works for one may not work for another. Experiment with different positions and techniques to find what works best for you and your partner.

Chapter 6

Sexual Positions

Sexual positions play a crucial role in sensual pleasure and satisfying your man in bed. Different positions offer varying degrees of sensations, intimacy, and control, allowing you to explore different facets of your sexuality. Whether you're after variety, deeper penetration, intimacy, or pleasure mastery, this chapter will guide you through the most popular sexual positions to make your sexual experiences more fulfilling.

Missionary Position

The missionary position is one of the classic sexual positions where the man is on top of the woman, facing her. It's ideal for intimate sex sessions, maintaining eye contact, and showing love and affection. The position also allows for deep penetration, which stimulates the G-spot and enables the woman to experience more powerful orgasms.

To perform this position, lie on your back and spread your legs slightly. Your partner slides in between your legs, supporting his weight on his elbows. You can wrap your legs around his waist, and he can place his hands on either side of your head for balance.

Pros: This position allows for intimacy, eye contact and deeper penetration.

Cons: It can be tiring for the man to support his weight for an extended period of time, and there is a lack of control and variety.

Tip: Try placing a pillow under your hips to change the angle of penetration and create new sensations.

Doggy Style

This position is all about power and dominance. The woman is on all fours with her hands and knees on the bed, while the man penetrates from behind. It allows for deep penetration and a unique angle that hits the G-spot for intense orgasms. Moreover, it creates visual excitement and stimulates the dominant and submissive dynamics of the couple.

To perform this position, kneel on all fours with your hands placed firmly on the bed. Your partner gets behind you, entering from the back. He can hold onto your hips for leverage and control the depth and speed of penetration.

Pros: It allows for deep penetration, hits the G-spot and creates a sense of domination and submission.

Cheryl Bach

Cons: The angle of penetration can be uncomfortable or even painful for some women, and it can be difficult to maintain a rhythm or connection.

Tip: Try shifting your weight back onto your partner, changing the angle of penetration and allowing for clitoral stimulation.

Cowgirl/Reverse Cowgirl

In this position, the woman is in control, with the man lying on his back. In the cowgirl position, the woman straddles the man, facing him, while in the reverse cowgirl, she faces away from him. This position allows for maximum clitoral stimulation, while also giving the woman control over the speed and depth of penetration. It also allows for deeper penetration and access to the G-spot.

To perform the cowgirl position, straddle your partner, placing your knees on either side of his body. Lean back slightly, using your arms for support as you ride him, controlling the rhythm and speed of penetration.

Pros: This position gives women control, while also allowing for maximum clitoral stimulation and deep penetration.

Cons: The lack of eye contact and intimacy may not be appealing to some couples.

Tip: Try leaning forward and placing your hands on your partner's chest for intimate eye contact, or try reversing the position for a new sensation.

Spooning

This position is ideal for cuddly, intimate sex sessions. The couple lies on their sides, with the man behind the woman.

Cheryl Bach

The woman can lift her top leg to allow for deeper penetration and more effective clitoral stimulation.

To perform this position, lie on your side facing away from your partner, with your knees bent. Your partner can then spoon you from behind, entering his penis into your vagina. You can adjust the angle of entry by shifting one or both legs, and your partner can place his hand on your hip for stability and deeper thrusting.

Pros: This is an intimate position that can be incredibly tender, and can allow for deep penetration and sensitive stimulation.

Cons: It can be difficult to maintain a rhythm, and it might not be ideal for those who prefer more active or adventurous sex positions.

Pleasure Mastery

Tip: Try incorporating a vibrator or dildo for extra stimulation.

Transitioning Between Positions

Transitioning between positions can be just as important as the positions themselves. Communication is essential when transitioning, as it helps prevent discomfort or pain. When transitioning between positions, try to maintain some level of physical contact to ensure the connection is not lost. You can move together to the next position, or take a break and switch things up gradually.

It's also important to ensure that both partners are comfortable and agree to the new position before transitioning. If either partner feels discomfort or non-consent, then it's better to make changes or stop completely.

Cheryl Bach

Takeaway

Sexual positions can open up new avenues of pleasure and connection with your partner, but it's important to choose positions that are comfortable and enjoyable for both partners. Experimenting is key, as each position offers different sensations and techniques. Remember, communication is key, so be sure to talk to your partner about what you both enjoy and want to explore. By combining different positions and communicating effectively, you can create a fulfilling and satisfying sexual experience.

Chapter 7

Experimentation

Experimentation is at the core of sexual pleasure and satisfaction. As you explore new activities and fantasies with your partner, you open up new avenues of pleasure and deepen the connection between you. This chapter will guide you through the importance of experimentation, exploring new activities, and how to talk about boundaries and consent.

Importance of Experimentation

Experimentation keeps the excitement and spark alive in a relationship. By exploring new activities and fantasies, you can discover new likes, dislikes, and preferences. It can help with communication and intimacy as it involves building trust and vulnerability. Both partners should feel comfortable and safe to talk about their desires and boundaries, regardless of their experience level.

Exploring New Activities, Fantasies and Role-Playing

1. Start by discussing your fantasies: Begin by talking with your partner about your secret fantasies and listening to theirs. This can be done in a casual and non-judgmental manner. Share what you imagine yourself doing, whether it's a specific position or activity. You can also talk about what you've seen in movies or read in books. Be open to exploring your partner's fantasies as well.

2. Try new things together: Once you have discussed your fantasies, agree to try out a few things together. Research new positions, techniques, or role-playing scenarios and select a few that you both want to try. Make sure to take the time to thoroughly explore and experiment with each new activity.

3. Take it slow: While exploration is important, it's equally important to take things slow. Gradually increase intensity rather than jumping right into the deep end. Start with something simple and build up as you start to feel more comfortable. Trying too much at once can be overwhelming and may lead to discomfort or negative experiences.

4. Build trust and intimacy: Experimentation is all about trust and intimacy, so make sure to create a loving and non-judgmental environment. It's essential to take the time to check in with each other throughout the process to ensure that both of you feel comfortable and satisfied with the activities you're trying out.

5. Incorporate toys and props: Toys and props can be great tools for experimentation as they can help enhance pleasure, intimacy, and creativity. Start by trying out a simple vibrator or a blindfold to explore new sensations. Pornography can also be helpful in identifying new

Cheryl Bach

positions or activities to try out, but be mindful not to make your partner uncomfortable in the process.

How to Talk About Boundaries and Consent

Discussing boundaries and consent before trying new activities is critical.

Here are some tips on how to have that conversation:

Set the Right Mood: Choose a neutral setting, where both of you can feel comfortable, and won't be disturbed, choose a time when both of you are relaxed.

Be Honest: Be transparent and honest about what you want and don't want to experiment with. Explain your boundaries and limits clearly.

Listen Actively: It's important to listen to your partner as much as you talk. Allow them to express their opinions and boundaries.

Respect their Decision: If your partner is hesitant to try something, then respect their decision. Do not push or pressure them into doing anything they do not feel comfortable with.

Establish a Safe Word: Establishing a safe word provides a way for either of you to communicate your discomfort or need for a break during sexual activity. The safe word should be a simple word or phrase that is easy to remember and not typically used during sex.

Get Consent: Remember to always seek consent from your partner before trying out any new activity. Consent should be given freely and enthusiastically, and it can always be withdrawn at any point during sexual activity.

Check-in: During sexual activity, you should always check in with your partner regularly to ensure that they are comfortable and enjoying themselves. If your partner has withdrawn their consent or no longer feels comfortable during an activity, stop immediately.

In conclusion, experimentation is key to a fulfilling and satisfying sexual experience. It allows for exploration of new activities, fantasies, and role-playing scenarios, helping to build trust, intimacy, and communication between partners. Remember to have open, honest communication when discussing your boundaries and desires and always seek consent and respect your partner's decisions.

Chapter 8

Orgasmic Mastery

For many men, the pinnacle of sexual pleasure is reaching orgasm. As a partner, your role in helping them achieve this goal can be incredibly rewarding and pleasurable. In this chapter, you will learn how to give your man the best orgasm possible. We will also explore the different types of orgasms men can experience, ways to stimulate the prostate for heightened pleasure, and techniques for building up to an intense orgasm.

How to Give Your Man the Best Orgasm Possible

Build up anticipation with foreplay: Foreplay is crucial in building anticipation and arousal. It's essential to take your time and touch your partner in such a way that builds up tension and excitement. Kiss, lick, and caress his sensitive areas to turn him on.

Communicate: Communication is key to understanding what your partner likes and dislikes in bed. Ask him what feels good, when to speed up, slow down or if he wants you to keep doing what you're doing. It's also important to pay attention to his body language during sex and respond accordingly. Nonverbal cues such as moaning, breathing patterns, and body movement can tell a lot about what he likes.

Experiment with different techniques: Every man is different with unique preferences, so it's important to experiment with different techniques to find out what works for your partner. Techniques such as oral sex, hand stimulation, and intercourse all have different sensations and can produce different orgasms.

Be observant: The more attentive you are to your partner's response, the easier it is to know when he is nearing orgasm. This is the moment when you want to focus on a particular technique that you know he loves and increase the pace and intensity.

Focus on his pleasure: During sex, focus your attention on your partner's pleasure rather than your own. This will enable you to connect with your partner and help him achieve the best orgasm possible.

Different Types of Orgasms Men can Experience

There are various kinds of orgasms men can experience, including:

Penile Orgasms: This is the most common type of orgasm in men and is achieved through stimulation of the penis during sex or masturbation.

Cheryl Bach

Prostate Orgasms: The prostate gland is a highly sensitive area in men and can be stimulated through anal penetration or massaging the external perineum.

Blended Orgasms: These orgasms occur when both the penis and prostate are stimulated simultaneously.

Full-Body Orgasms: These orgasms occur when the entire body experiences intense pleasure and muscle contractions during ejaculation. They usually require prolonged sexual stimulation and are rare but highly satisfying.

Tips on How to Stimulate the Prostate for Heightened Pleasure

The prostate gland is a highly sensitive area that can provide intense pleasure when stimulated correctly.

Here are some tips on how to stimulate the prostate for heightened pleasure:

Pleasure Mastery

Start slow: Always start slowly and gently, especially if your partner has never experienced prostate stimulation before. Use plenty of lube and communicate with him to make sure he is comfortable and enjoying the experience.

Use fingers or toys: You can use your fingers or toys designed for prostate stimulation to achieve this. Toys such as butt plugs and prostate massagers are perfect for exploring prostate stimulation.

Experiment with different positions: There are several comfortable positions for prostate stimulation. One basic position is having your partner lie on his back with a pillow under his hips to expose the perineum and prostate area.

Combine with other forms of stimulation: Prostate stimulation can be more pleasurable when combined with other forms of sexual stimulation such as oral sex or hand stimulation.

Techniques for Building Up to an Intense Orgasm

Building up to an intense orgasm is all about gradually increasing pleasure and avoiding over-stimulation.

Here are some techniques that you can use to achieve this:

Edging: Edging is a technique where you bring your partner close to orgasm, then pull back and start over again. This cycle of building up and slowing down can lead to an intense orgasm.

Kegels: Kegel exercises can help men achieve stronger orgasms by strengthening the pelvic floor muscles. The stronger these muscles are, the more powerful the contractions during orgasm.

Deep breathing: Deep breathing techniques, such as belly breathing can help men relax during sex. This can increase blood flow to the penis and improve overall sexual performance, leading to a more intense orgasm.

Mutual masturbation: Mutual masturbation is where you and your partner stimulate each other manually or orally. This technique allows you to learn what your partner likes and how they respond to certain forms of stimulation, making it easier to build up to an intense orgasm.

In conclusion, mastering the art of giving your man an intense orgasm requires practice, patience, communication, and experimentation. Remember, every man is different, and what works for one may not work for another. Understanding his unique needs, experimenting with different techniques, and communicating frequently with him is key to giving him the best orgasm possible. With time and practice, you'll become an expert in orgasmic mastery, and your partner will thank you for the unforgettable sexual experiences you'll be able to provide. Don't be afraid to explore new methods like prostate stimulation or mutual masturbation to heighten pleasure and achieve an intense orgasm. Focus on building anticipation, experimenting with different techniques, and paying close attention to your partner's cues. And always remember to communicate openly and honestly. With these tips, you can become a master at giving your man an unforgettable orgasmic experience.

Chapter 9

Post-Sex

Congratulations, you've just given your man an amazing orgasm! Now what? While many couples focus on the act of sex itself, many forget the crucial importance of post-sex intimacy and aftercare. In this chapter, we will explore why post-sex intimacy is important, techniques on how to cuddle, and the role of aftercare in keeping your connection strong.

The Importance of Post-Sex Intimacy

Post-sex intimacy refers to the time you spend cuddling, talking, or spending quality time with your partner after sex. This time is crucial, as it helps promote emotional bonding and helps to deepen your connection with your partner. Many people believe that intimacy ends with ejaculation, but that couldn't be further from the truth. In fact, intimacy can help intensify the pleasure of sex and create long-lasting memories.

Cuddling Techniques

Cuddling is one way to promote intimacy and deepen your connection with your partner.

Here are a few techniques to help you master the art of cuddling:

Spooning: This is perhaps the most classic cuddling position, which is why it deserves first mention. The larger partner can take up the role of the "big spoon" and wrap their arm around the "little spoon," providing them with a sense of comfort and security. It's important to note that this doesn't always have to be a man-woman dynamic and can vary depending on individual relationships.

Face-to-face: In this position, both partners are facing each other, holding each other close, and looking into each other's eyes. This position can help promote intimacy and create deeper emotional connections between partners.

Leg entanglement: This is a cozy and intimate way of cuddling where partners entangle their legs together. This position can create feelings of closeness and bonding that not only helps in physical intimacy but also strengthens emotional connection.

Head on chest: This is a classic cuddling position where one partner rests their head on the other partner's chest. The partner providing the cushioning support usually places their hand over their partner's shoulder or gently strokes their hair.

The Role of Aftercare

Aftercare refers to the care provided to a partner after sex. This care is important, as it helps ensure that both partners feel safe, respected, and valued.

Here are some ways to provide aftercare to your partner:

Communicate: After sex, it's important to communicate with your partner and ask how they're feeling. Make sure they feel comfortable and ask if there's anything you can do to make them feel more comfortable or taken care of.

Hydrate: Sex can take a lot of energy, and it's important that both partners stay hydrated. Offer your partner some water or other hydrating fluids to help them replenish their energy.

Snuggle up: Cuddle with your partner, ensuring that they feel safe and comfortable enough to fall asleep. Show them that their comfort is a top priority for you.

Take care of each other: If your partner needs extra attention or care in any way, such as by applying a warm compress or affectionately placing a hand on their back, make sure you provide it. This can help your partner feel valued, appreciated and cared for in moments that are intimate, vulnerable and critical for any relationship.

In conclusion, post-sex intimacy and aftercare are crucial parts of any intimate encounter. It's important to remember that while sex is a physical act, it has emotional and mental repercussions as well. By engaging in post-sex intimacy, you can deepen your connection with your partner, show them that they are valued, and ensure that both of you feel cared for and respected.

Being able to master the art of cuddling, providing aftercare, and engaging in post-sex intimacy are all ways to promote a strong and healthy relationship that is satisfying for both partners. Remember, intimacy is not just about sex; it's about creating an emotional bond and touch has the ability to heal, love and provide security.

Pleasure Mastery

Chapter 10

Maintenance

Now that you've mastered the art of giving your man pleasure in bed, it's time to focus on the importance of maintenance in keeping the spark alive in your relationship. In this chapter, we will explore why maintaining intimacy is crucial, techniques for incorporating pleasure and intimacy into your daily routine, and encouragement to continue exploring and experimenting with each other.

The Importance of Maintenance

Many couples make the mistake of assuming that the effort put into their sex life during the early stages of their relationship should be enough to carry them through their entire lives together. However, a healthy and rewarding sex life requires ongoing maintenance to sustain it over the long term.

It's important to remember that life can get in the way, that stress, work, and other commitments can undermine your desire, satisfaction and connection as a couple but putting in the effort to maintain intimacy can help keep the spark alive. By making intimacy and pleasure a priority in your relationship, you are investing in your emotional and physical well-being and the well-being of your partner.

Incorporating Pleasure and Intimacy into Your Daily Routine

One way to maintain intimacy is by incorporating pleasure and intimacy into your daily routine. This can help keep the connection fresh and exciting, even outside the bedroom.

Here are some techniques to try:

Small gestures: Make small gestures that show your partner that you care about them and are thinking of them throughout the day. It could be as simple as sending a flirty text message or leaving a sweet note for them to find.

Set aside time for intimacy: Making time for intimacy is essential, especially if you have a busy schedule. Setting aside even just 15 minutes a day to connect physically and emotionally with your partner can make a big difference in maintaining intimacy. Use this time to chat, cuddle, or engage in any type of sexual activity that feels right for both of you.

Date nights: Plan regular date nights with your partner to spice things up and keep the spark alive. Whether it's a fancy dinner or a night out at the movies, make sure to prioritize this time together.

Experiment: Don't be afraid to experiment with different sexual techniques or try new things in the bedroom. This can help keep the passion alive and prevent things from becoming routine. Remember that every person is different, and being open to exploring each other's bodies and desires is key to maintaining intimacy in the long term.

Encouragement to Continue Exploring and Experimenting with Each Other

Finally, it's important to encourage each other to continue exploring and experimenting with each other. This can help you discover new ways to give each other pleasure and keep things fresh and exciting in the bedroom.

Remember, exploring and experimenting should always be done with mutual respect and consent. Communication is important in any healthy sexual relationship, and talking openly about your desires and boundaries can help make sure that both partners feel safe and fulfilled.

It's also important to stay open-minded and flexible in your approach to sex. Sometimes things may not go exactly as planned, but staying positive and open to new experiences can help you find pleasure in unexpected ways.

In conclusion, maintaining the spark in your relationship takes effort and ongoing maintenance, but it's worth it for a healthy and rewarding sex life. By incorporating pleasure and intimacy into your daily routine, exploring and experimenting with each other, and making intimacy a priority, you can keep the passion alive for years to come. Remember to communicate with your partner openly and honestly, and be willing to try new things to keep things fresh and exciting.

Maintenance is not just about keeping the spark alive in your relationship, it's about creating a healthy, sustainable, and fulfilling sexual relationship with your partner. When you prioritize intimacy and pleasure in your relationship, you are investing in the emotional and physical well-being of each other and nurturing a deep and loving connection that will last a lifetime.

So take the time to maintain your relationship, explore and experiment with each other, and always keep the lines of communication open. With the right attitude and approach, you can have an amazing, fulfilling, and passionate sex life for years to come.

Conclusion

Congratulations, you've made it to the end of "Pleasure Mastery: An Ultimate Guide to Satisfying Your Man in Bed"! In this book, we've explored a variety of techniques and strategies for enhancing your sexual pleasure and satisfaction, and building a deep and fulfilling connection with your partner.

Recap of Key Points

Let's do a quick recap of the key points from this book:

Communication is Key: Communicating openly and honestly with your partner is essential for a healthy and satisfying sexual relationship.

Self-Exploration: Understanding your own body and what feels good to you is crucial for knowing how to communicate your desires and needs to your partner.

Techniques for Pleasure: We've discussed a variety of techniques for enhancing pleasure, including foreplay, oral sex, different sex positions, and

Embracing Your Desires: Don't be afraid to explore and embrace your desires, even if they may seem taboo or unconventional.

Consensual Experimentation: Experimenting with your partner can help you both discover new ways to experience pleasure, but it's important to always communicate and respect each other's boundaries.

Taking Control of Your Pleasure: Taking the time to prioritize your own sexual pleasure and satisfaction can lead to a more fulfilling connection with your partner.

Final Words of Encouragement to Take Control of Your Sexual Pleasure

As you continue to explore your own sexuality and journey towards pleasure mastery, remember to stay open-minded,

Cheryl Bach

communicate with your partner, and never be afraid to ask for what you want. Each person's sexual experiences and preferences are unique, so take the time to explore and experiment until you find what works best for you and your partner.

In conclusion, we hope that this book has inspired you to take control of your sexual pleasure and explore new ways to experience intimacy with your partner. With the right mindset and techniques, you can achieve ultimate satisfaction and create a deep and lasting connection with your loved one.

Bonus Material on Other Resources to Further Explore Sexual Pleasure and Connection

But our journey doesn't have to end here. There are many other resources available for further exploration of sexual pleasure and connection.

Pleasure Mastery

Here are some bonus materials to get you started:

Educational Resources: Books, websites, and classes can provide valuable insights into sexual health, pleasure, and communication.

Sex Toys: Sex toys can be a fun and exciting way to explore new sensations and enhance your pleasure.

Communication Tools: Apps and games designed to promote communication between partners can help build trust, intimacy, and deepen your connection.

Remember that every person's journey towards pleasure mastery is unique, so don't feel pressure to conform to any specific standards or expectations. Take the time to explore and experiment with what feels good for you and your partner while always maintaining mutual respect and consent.

In conclusion, we want to encourage you to continue exploring and mastering your sexual pleasure. Embrace your desires, communicate openly with your partner, and remember that pleasure is not a destination but a lifelong journey.

We hope this book has been helpful in guiding you towards sexual pleasure mastery and sparking new ideas for enhancing intimacy with your partner. Remember to prioritize your pleasure and never stop exploring new ways to experience sexual satisfaction and connection.

May your journey towards pleasure mastery be fulfilling and exciting!

www.ingramcontent.com/pod-product-compliance
Lightning Source LLC
Chambersburg PA
CBHW051835250726
48659CB00005B/1851